Marwa Gargouri
Hela Gargouri
Tlil Ahmed

Covid-19 infection among healthcare workers in Gabès

Marwa Gargouri
Hela Gargouri
Tlil Ahmed

Covid-19 infection among healthcare workers in Gabès

Clinico-biological study of Covid-19 infection in healthcare workers at the university hospital in Gabés

Imprint

Any brand names and product names mentioned in this book are subject to trademark, brand or patent protection and are trademarks or registered trademarks of their respective holders. The use of brand names, product names, common names, trade names, product descriptions etc. even without a particular marking in this work is in no way to be construed to mean that such names may be regarded as unrestricted in respect of trademark and brand protection legislation and could thus be used by anyone.

Cover image: www.ingimage.com

This book is a translation from the original published under ISBN 978-620-6-71227-5.

Publisher:
Sciencia Scripts
is a trademark of
Dodo Books Indian Ocean Ltd. and OmniScriptum S.R.L publishing group

120 High Road, East Finchley, London, N2 9ED, United Kingdom
Str. Armeneasca 28/1, office 1, Chisinau MD-2012, Republic of Moldova, Europe
Printed at: see last page
ISBN: 978-620-7-61550-6

CONTENTS

INTRODUCTION

Coronavirus 2019 (COVID-19) is an infectious disease caused by the SARS-COV-2 virus identified for the first time in China on 7 January 2020. The first cases have been reported since 31 December 2019 in the city of Wuhan [1]. On 30/01/2020, the World Health Organisation (WHO) declared the SARS-COV-2 epidemic a public health emergency of international concern [2]. Then after rapid spread and acceleration of cases worldwide, the WHO officially declared the COVID-19 outbreak a pandemic on 11 March 2020. [3].

Infection with SARS-COV-2 is a polymorphous disease. The majority of people infected with COVID-19 will experience only mild or moderate symptoms and will recover without any particular treatment, but some will become seriously ill and require medical attention.With the number of cases of infection on the rise worldwide, COVID-19 has become the talk of the town these days. Indeed, when we look at the people affected by this pandemic, we find that healthcare workers occupy first place, as the population of workers at increased risk of developing an infection due to their occupational exposure. Throughout the world, healthcare workers have been particularly affected by COVID-19. In China, 3.8% of cases were among HCWs, compared with 18% in France, 17% in Ontario, 16% in Spain and the United States, and 12% in Italy and Germany. In Quebec, as of June 14, 2020, 13,581 (25%) of the 54,054 confirmed cases in Quebec were identified as TdeS. [4]

In Tunisia, the first case was a man arriving from Italy on 27 February 2020 and hospitalised on 3 March 2020. By 10 May 2022, 396,000 COVID-19-positive cases had been recorded in Tunisia, including 1,515 deaths [5].

Health professionals had a higher risk of coronavirus infection than the general population. This is why we focused on these workers, limiting our study to the University Hospital of Gabès.

RESEARCH OBJECTIVES

In order to carry out this work, the following objectives have been set:

• To study the epidemiology and characteristics of SARS-COV2 infection in healthcare workers at the University Hospital of Gabés.

• Describe the management of protective measures and their use by healthcare staff

• Give some solutions to avoid, in the event of a new wave, the constraints found during previous crises.

MATERIALS AND METHODS

I. Search quote :

This is a cross-sectional descriptive study including the hospital's healthcare staff.University of Gabes. In the course of this study, the members interviewed answered our questionnaire personally and anonymously.

II. Study environment and period :

This study was carried out at the University Hospital of Gabès during the months of April and October. May 2022. The departments included in our study were the following:

▶ Pneumology Department

▶ Infectious Diseases Department

▶ Cardiology department

▶ Medicine department

▶ Women's and men's surgery department

▶ Emergency service

▶ SAMU

▶ Radiology

▶ Laboratory

III. The study population :

For this study, we selected a population of 100 healthcare workers working at the University Hospital of Gabes in the departments most likely to be in contact with confirmed or suspected Covid_19 patients. :

- Emergency service: 21

- Laboratory:12

- Infectious diseases department: 11

- Cardiology department: 10

- Medical department: 10

- Pneumology department: 9

- Radiology:8

- SAMU: 7

- Women's surgery department :6

- Male surgery department :6

IV. Inclusion and exclusion criteria :

1. Inclusion criteria :

- Care staff with the grade of: doctor, nurse, technician, worker

- Staff working in the Pneumology, Infectious Diseases, Cardiology, Medicine, Male and Female Surgery, Emergency, EMS, Laboratory and Radiology departments.

- The choice of these services was based on the significant risk of transmission of COVID-.

19. It includes the COVID circuit, including the emergency department, the EMS, the radiology department for thoracic CT scans and the laboratory department for COVID-19 tests and PCRs, as well as the referral departments for pneumology, infectious diseases, cardiology, medicine and surgery.

2. Exclusion criteria :

- The refusal declared by certain healthcare staff.

- Staff working in other departments.

- Absence of certain staff during our study period.

V. Data collection :

This study was carried out by means of a questionnaire consisting of 30 questions (identification part: comprising 6 questions, 4 open questions and 20 closed questions) targeted at 100 healthcare staff working at the University Hospital of Gabes.

VI. Data collection process :

We went to the 10 departments to inform potential staff about the study (context and objectives). We then distributed the questionnaire to those who agreed to take part. Each staff member spent an average of 15 minutes answering the various parts of the questionnaire.

VII. Data capture and analysis :

The data is collected manually.

Data was entered using computer equipment (2 computers), typed in Microsoft Office Word 2007 and processed using Microsoft Office Excel 2007.

The results are presented using Excel and Word.

ANALYSIS AND RESULTS

I. Socio-demographic data :

1. Gender :

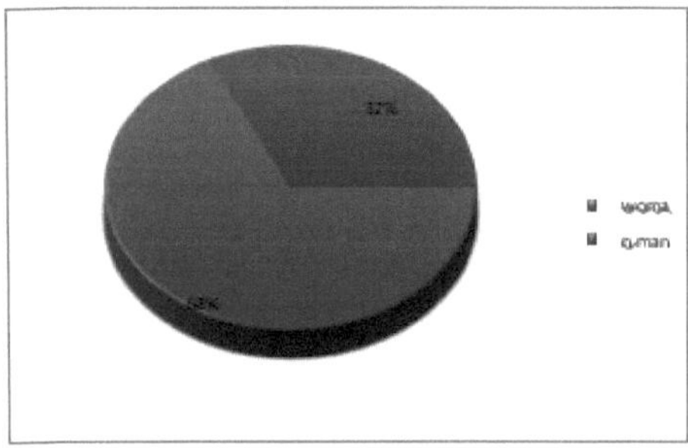

Figure 1: Breakdown of staff by gender

- The majority of the population studied is made up of women (68%).

2. Age :

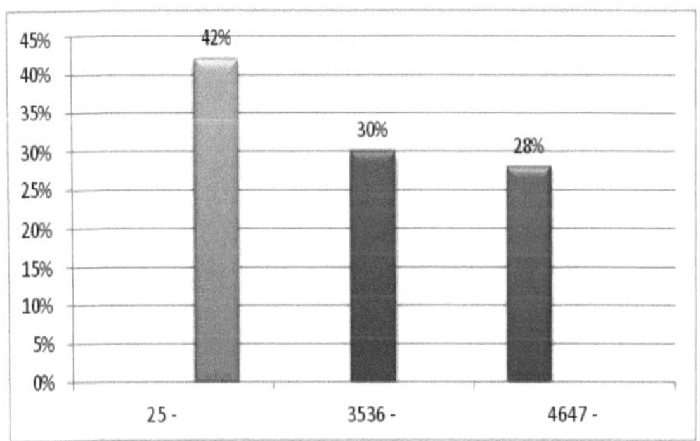

Figure 2: Breakdown of staff by age

- Participants' ages range from a high of 57 to a low of around 25. Almost half the population is in the 25-35 age bracket (42%).

3. History :

Table I: Breakdown of staff by antecedents

	Workforce	Percentage
No previous history	42	42%
Surgical history	25	25%
Hypertension	13	13%
Diabetes	11	11%
Other	8	8%
Chronic lung disease	4	4%

• Almost half the population had no medical or surgical history.

4. The profession :

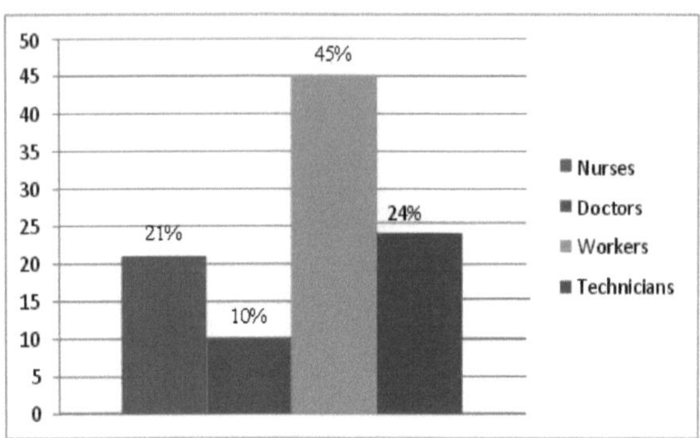

Figure 3: Breakdown of staff by profession

• The majority of staff interviewed were nurses (45%). The remainder were 24% doctors, 21% technicians and 10% manual workers.

5. Length of service :

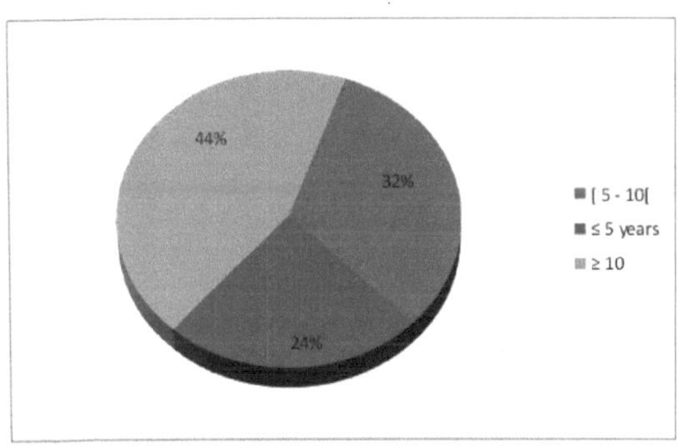

Figure 4: Breakdown of staff by length of service

• The majority of staff surveyed (44%) have been with the company for more than 10 years.

6. Work department :

Table II: Breakdown of staff by department

Work department	Workforce	Percentage
Emergency service	21	21%
Laboratory	12	12%
Infectious diseases department	11	11%
Cardiology department	10	10%
Medicine department	10	10%
Pneumology Department	9	9%
Radiology	8	8%
SAMU	7	7%
Women's surgery	6	6%
Men's surgery	6	6%
Total	100	100%

• The staff surveyed in our population are spread across 10 departments with very similar staffing levels.

• The majority of participants worked in emergency departments (21%).

II. Experience and management of illness :

1. History of COVID-19 disease :

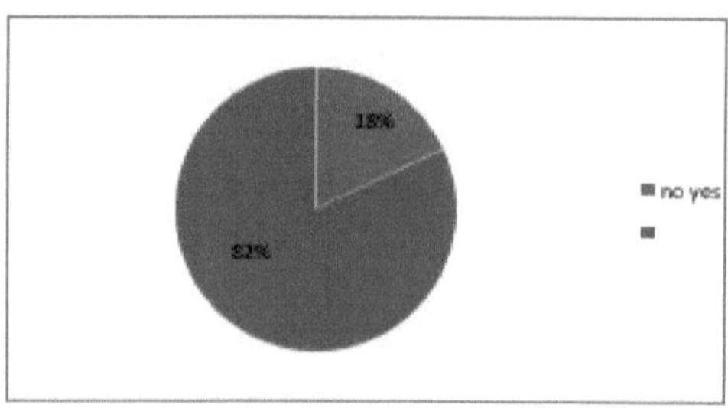

Figure 5: Breakdown of staff by history of illness in the COVID-19

• In our study, the majority of the population (82%) contracted COVID-19.

2. Breakdown of staff by number of times sick by COVID-19:

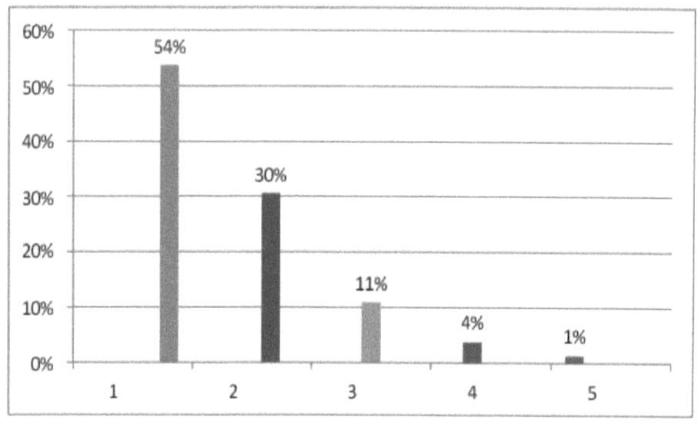

Figure 6: Breakdown of staff by number of times sickened by COVID-19

• Most participants (54%) were affected only once by COVID-19, while 1% were affected 5 times.

3. The symptoms of the disease present in the participants :

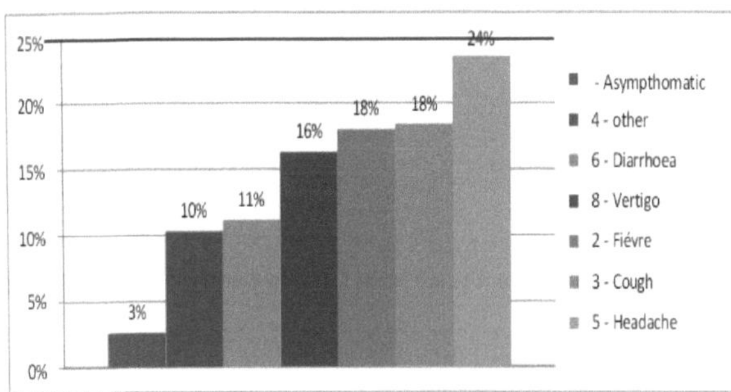

Figure 7: Breakdown of staff by symptoms of this pandemic

• In our study, the most common signs were headache (24%) and cough and fever (18%). Approximately 3% of the subjects interviewed had no symptoms.

4. The method for confirming the diagnosis of infection by COVID-19 :

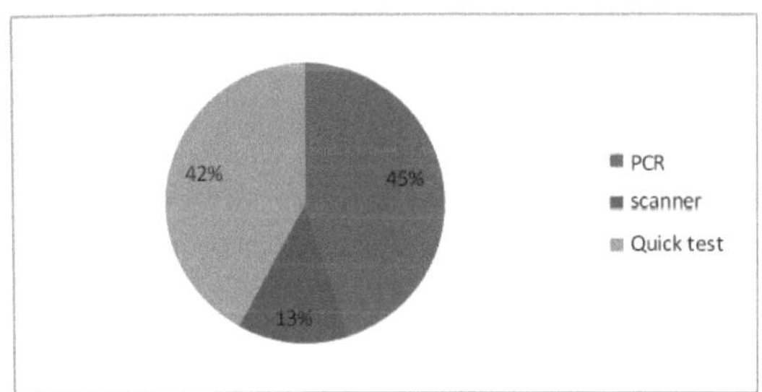

Figure 8: Breakdown of staff by confirmatory examination for disease

• Confirmation of the diagnosis of COVID-19 infection was based essentially on PCR (45%) and the SARS COV2 rapid test (42%).

5. Type of consultation :

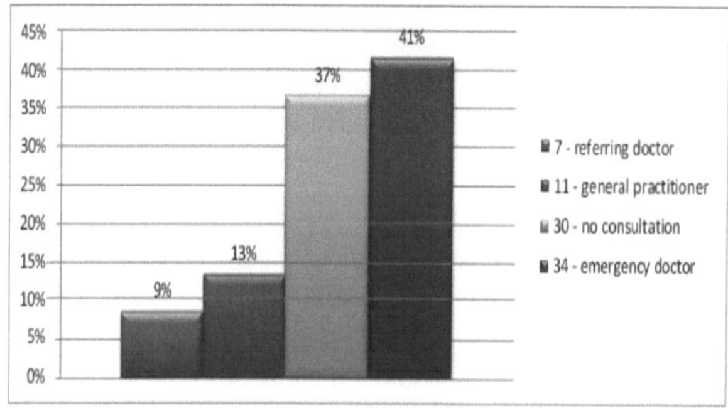

Figure 9: Breakdown of staff by type of consultation

• According to these results, almost half of the population confirmed the infection through an emergency doctor (41%).

6. Duration of symptoms :

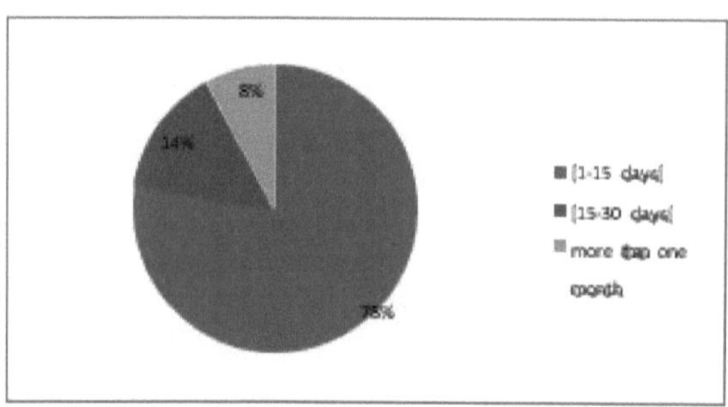

Figure 10: Breakdown of staff by duration of symptoms

• The majority of the population studied (78%) had persistent symptoms lasting from 1 to 15 days.

7. Time to return to work after infection with SARS COV2 :

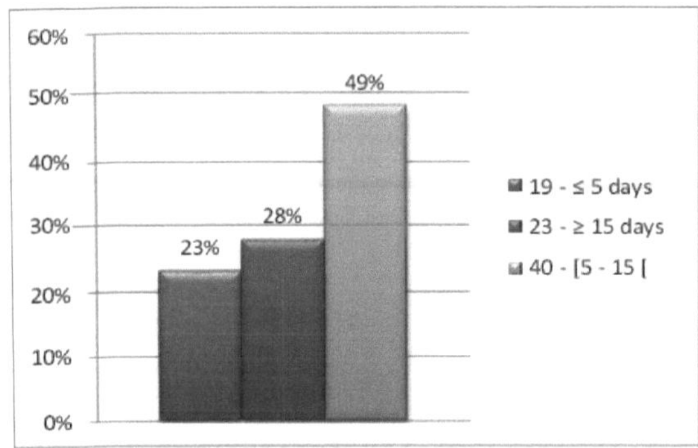

Figure 11: Breakdown of employees by time to return to work

• For most staff (49%), the time taken to return to work was between 5 and 15 days.

8. The persistence of disease symptoms after recovery :

a. The after-effects of the disease :

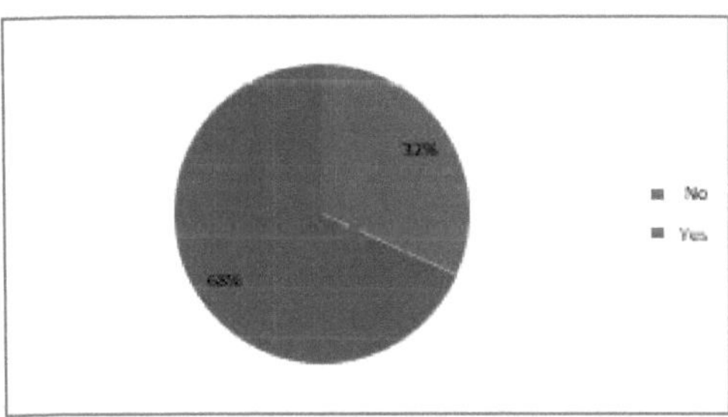

Figure 12: Distribution of staff according to the presence of after-effects.

• In our study, 68% of staff showed symptoms after recovery.

b. The breakdown according to the various after-effects :

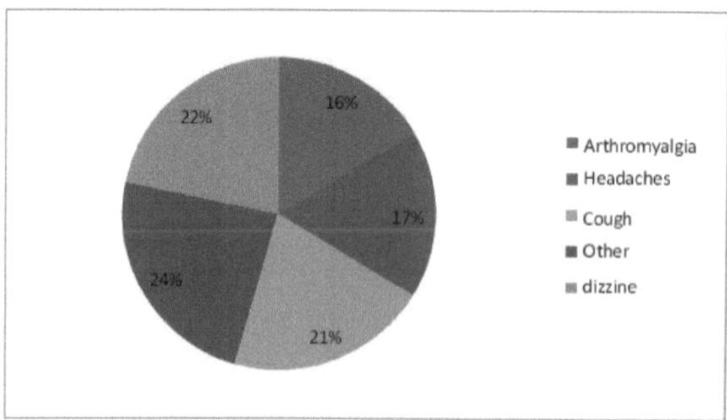

Figure 13: The different symptoms shown after recovery.

• A percentage of 68% was separated to different symptoms, among those that represented more than 41% of a total of 68 people (68% on 100% of the personnel that represented after-effects).

9. The nature of the management of the clinical picture :

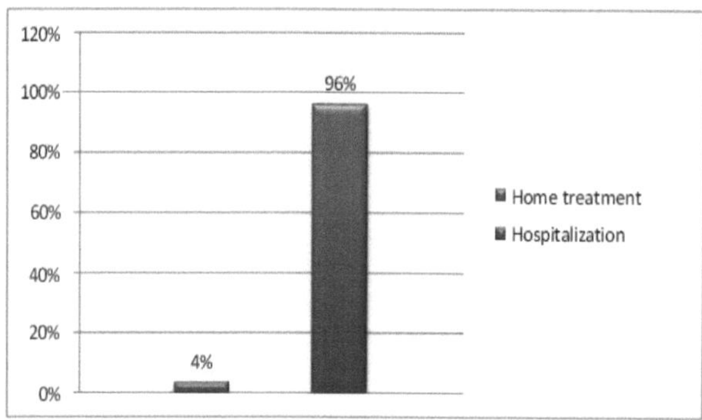

Figure 14: Breakdown of participants by type of care during illness

• Most of the population (96%) were treated at home and only 4% of participants required hospitalisation.

10. Compliance with containment :

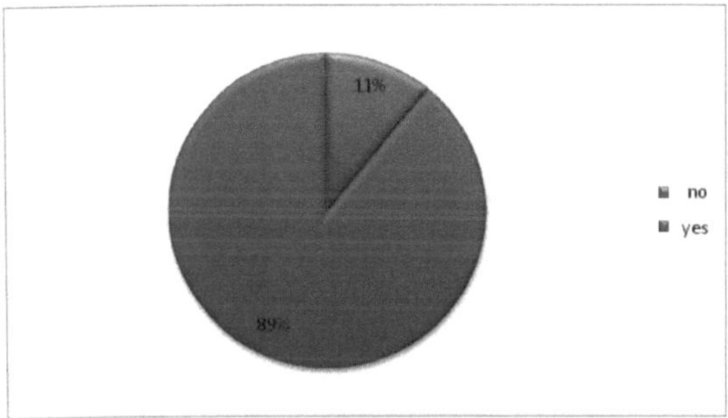

Figure 15: Breakdown of staff according to compliance with containment requirements

• It can be seen that the majority of staff questioned (89%) had complied appropriately with containment.

11. Type of treatment taken :

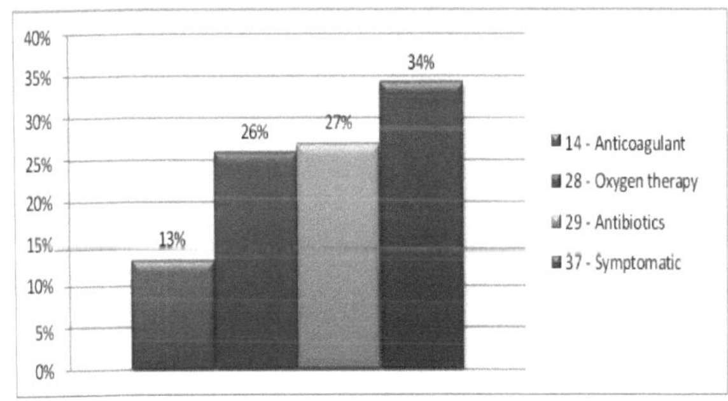

Figure 16: Breakdown of staff by type of treatment taken

• According to these results, all types of treatment were taken by staff, mainly symptomatic treatments (antipyretics, analgesics).

12. The mode of contamination :

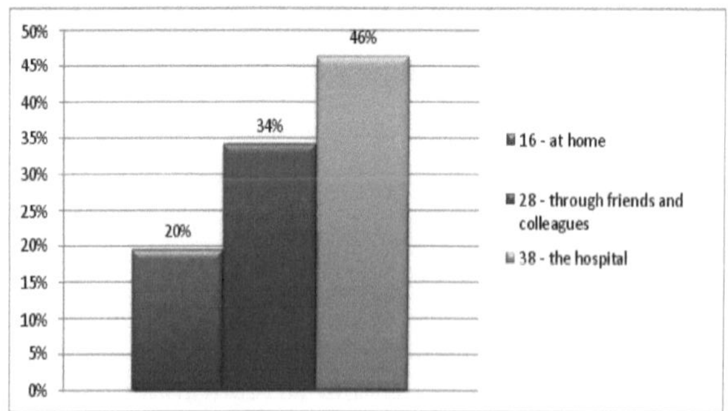

Figure 17: Breakdown of staff by mode of contamination

• The mode of contamination was mainly suffered in hospital (46%).

13. Infection of a member of the family and/or friends colleagues) :

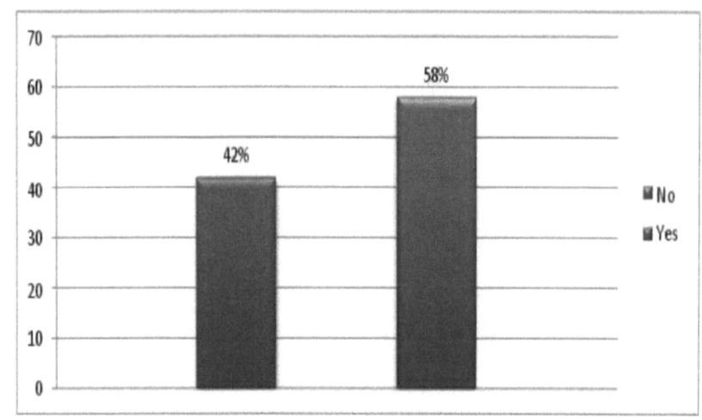

Figure 18: Breakdown of the population according to contamination in close contacts

• Almost half the population (42 people) had passed the disease on to their loved ones.

14. Vaccination against COVID -19 :

a. The number of people vaccinated :

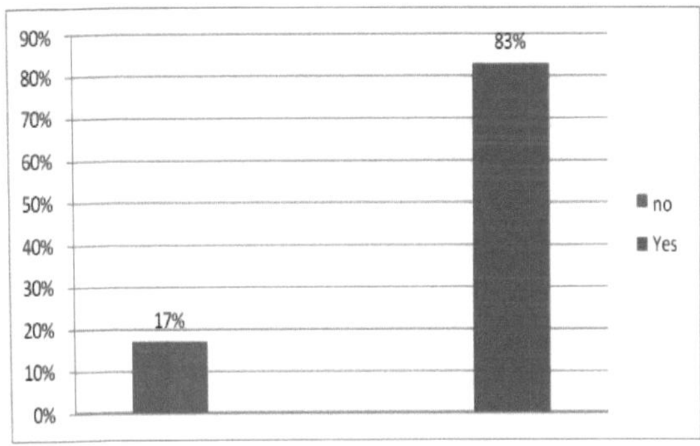

Figure 19: Breakdown of staff by type of COVID-19 vaccine taken.

More than two-thirds (83%) of the population studied had been vaccinated.

b. The type of vaccine most commonly used :

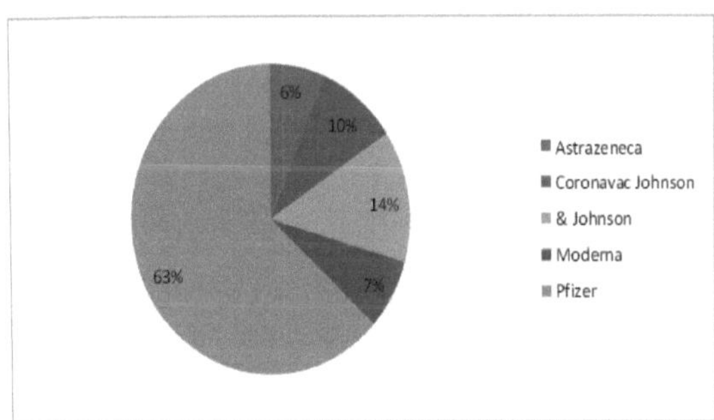

Figure 20: Breakdown of staff by type of vaccine

More than half the participants take Pfizer as a vaccine against covid- 19.

15. Distribution of staff according to the presence of deaths caused by t h e COVID-19 epidemic in the participants' entourage :

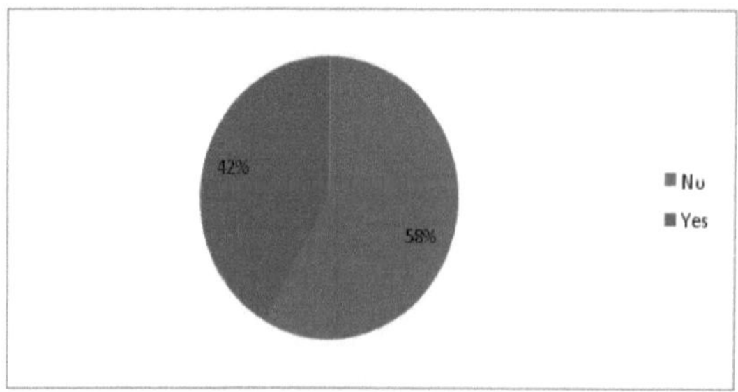

Figure 21: Distribution of staff according to the presence of deaths caused by COVID-19 in their entourage

- More than half of the population (58%) have died from the COVID-19 epidemic.

III. Protective measures against covid_19 and their application in hospital departments :

1. The distribution of protection measures :

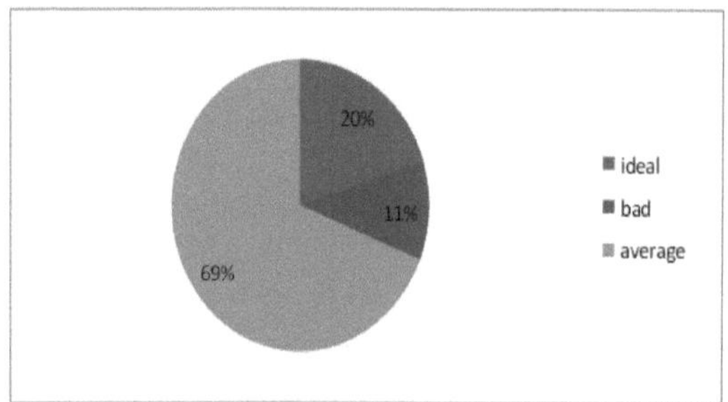

Figure 22: Distribution of protection measures within hospital departments

- Of the services studied, 69% had an average distribution.

2. Types of masks used :

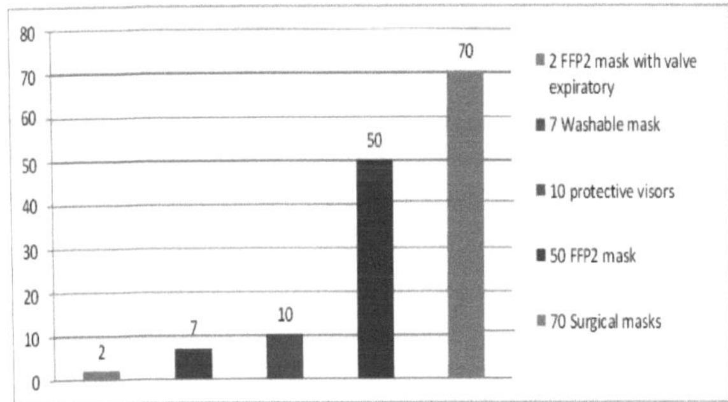

Figure 23: Types of mask used when working with patients

- The majority of staff questioned (70 out of 100) 70% used surgical masks when working in contact with patients.

3. The maximum time limit for using a single mask is :

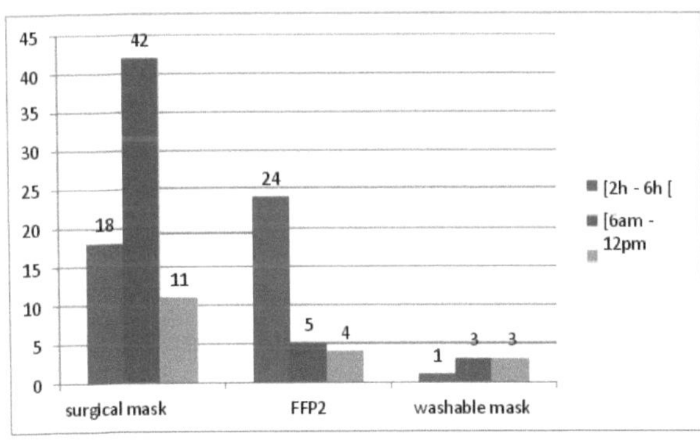

Figure 24: Staff responses on the maximum time required to use a single mask

- With regard to the use of surgical masks (the type most commonly used), the maximum delay for most staff is between 6 and 12 hours.
- Most people use FFP2 masks between 2 and 6 hours.

• As for washable masks (the type least used), staff use them between one and 3 days.

4. Barrier gestures :

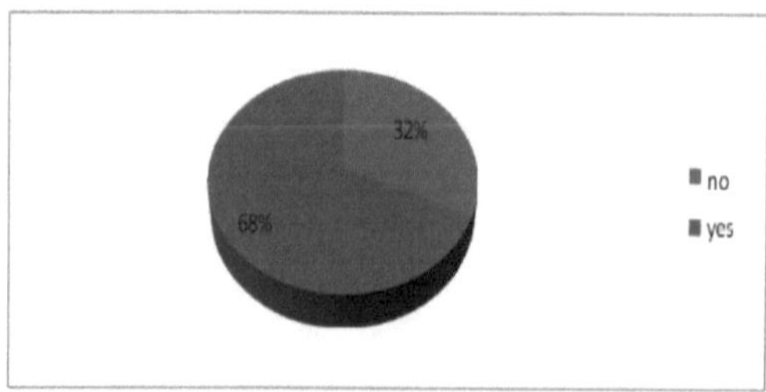

Figure 25: The service safety process and barrier actions.

• Sixty-eight per cent of the services selected emphasised barrier measures for staff, patients, carers and visitors.

5. Protection measures :

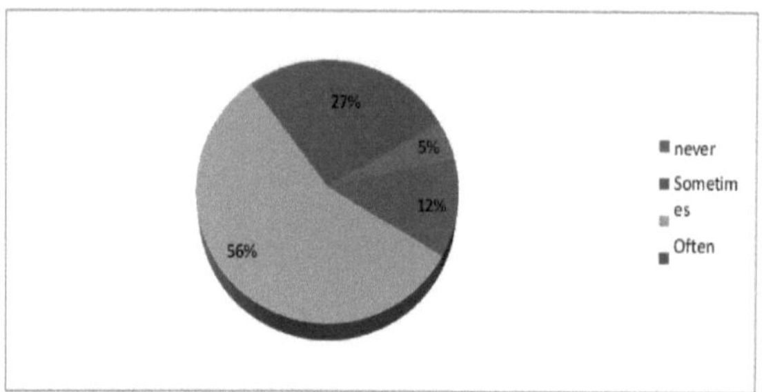

Figure 26: Compliance with colleague protection measures

• Five per cent of staff said that their colleagues never wore masks either in or out of hospital.

6. Time and space distribution :

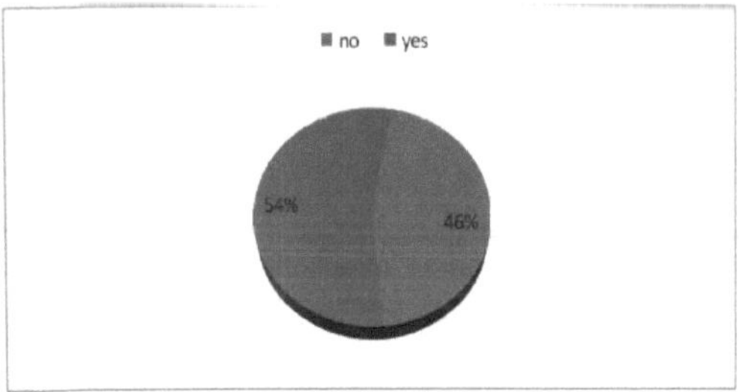

Figure 27: Time and space distribution in the workplace

• More than half of our customers feel that the time and space allocation is well suited to limiting congestion.

IV. Evaluation of precautionary measures and the psychological impact of covid-19 on healthcare workers :

• According to staff responses, our people have never ceased to be aware of the need to combat covid-19 and to take the necessary precautions in common areas of the hospital and in areas outside the hospital.

• There is a significant psychological impact caused by this pandemic (49% of participants confirm this negative impact on their psychology).

• With regard to the vaccine, most of the population (47%) confirmed that the symptoms had become less dangerous, and more than half of them had kept up their barrier measures even after vaccination.

1 : no, not at all2 : no, rather not3 : yes, rather4 : yes, completely

Table III: Evaluation of precautionary measures and psychological impact by the Covid- 19 among healthcare workers

	1	2	3	4
The preventive measures applied by health personnel are respected on the premises hospital common areas (rest room, cloakroom, etc.), buvette).	11%	20%	37%	32%
For patients presenting with symptoms atypical, protective measures against covid 19 are respected	21%	39%	26%	14%
Hospital staff occasionally wear masks in extra-hospital premises (the supermarkets, restaurants, etc.)	18%	40%	26%	16%
During this epidemic, visiting relatives remains frequent as usual.	22%	21%	20%	37%
This covid-19 pandemic is having an impact It is also a major psychological cause of suffering and uncertainty among staff health	13%	15%	25%	49%
Thanks to the effects of the vaccine, the symptoms are less dangerous and severe forms are less frequent.	13%	15%	25%	47%
less frequent.				
After vaccination, you need to keep up the barriers (masks, hydroalcoholic gel),	10%	10%	12%	68%

distancing) _

DISCUSSION

The health crisis was both sudden and exceptionally long-lasting, putting the health system at risk. hospital to a very high and unprecedented level of tension [6].Since the outbreak of the pandemic, healthcare workers have been the first line of defence against SARS-COV-2. As a result, they are exposed to a number of challenges: exhaustion, difficult patient triage, family separation and stigmatisation [7]. The subject of our work was covid_19 infection among health workers at the University Hospital of Gabès. Our study was based on a questionnaire sent to 100 healthcare workers, in order to assess the characteristics of this infection and the management and use of protective equipment.

I. Demographics :

During the study period, 100 staff were included. The sex ratio was 0.47, with a predominance of women (68%). This predominance was also marked in a study carried out including 135 health professionals working in COVID-19 health monitoring units in Morocco (a female predominance of 57.0% with a sex ratio of 1.32). While in a descriptive study done in the city of Debretabor (Ethiopia), among 183 healthcare workers participated in the survey, 67.76% of the participants were men. [8]

In our study, 42% of the staff questioned were aged between 25 and 35. A predominance of 70.4% aged over 40 was found in the study carried out in Morocco. In the same study, nurses represented only 14.8% of the population studied [9]. However, in our study, the majority were nurses (45%) When classified by seniority, the remarkable majority were those with more than 10 years' seniority (44%). On the other hand, the results obtained in a survey carried out in England showed that more than two thirds of 158 healthcare workers had been qualified for more than ten years. [10]

With regard to the history of this study population, it was found that the majority (42%) had no notable history. However, 50% had a history of hypertension, diabetes and chronic lung disease. This is similar to a similar study involving 430 healthcare workers in Nabeul (diabetes (8 cases), arterial hypertension (6 cases), and obesity (7 cases) [11]. Our targeted questionnaire for 100 people was distributed to 10 departments of the University Hospital of Gabés (Pneumology, Infectious Diseases, Cardiology, Medicine, Women's and Men's Surgery, Microbiology, Emergency, SAMU and Radiology), which appear to us to be the departments most directly or indirectly concerned by SARS COV2 disease. Among these departments, the emergency department presented the majority of our population (21%), which is not consistent with the results found in Cameron with a slight percentage of 3.3% [12].

II. Experience and management of illness :

Based on our study of the management of the COVID19 crisis at the University Hospital of Gabès, we focused on the experiences of health workers and the management of the disease during this pandemic.

1. Experience of illness :

In our study, we found that 82 staff had contracted COVID19, 69% of whom were female. These results are almost in line with those of the study carried out at a university hospital in Italy, where, out of 64 carers who contracted covid19, 43 (67.2%) were women [13]. In addition, 46% of those questioned had contracted the disease more than once. In a similar study carried out during the first and second waves in Paris on a sample of patients, 3 out of 7 people had contracted covid more than once (43%) [14]. These results showed that the recurrence of this disease does not only affect health professionals but also patients in almost equal measure, despite the fact that staff were more protected in terms of preventive measures. Of the staff questioned, a slight 6% were asymptomatic. This figure was 27.4% in a similar study carried out at Nabeul Regional Hospital [11].

In the same study, in 72.6% of symptomatic patients, the most frequent clinical signs were fever (61.2%), dry cough (30.6%) and fatigue (41.9%). Anosmia and agueusia were less frequent, observed respectively in 29% of patients. and 24% [11]. In our study, the most common clinical signs were headache (24%), fever (18%), cough (18%), dizziness (16%) and diarrhoea (11%). The average time to onset of these symptoms was between 1 and 15 days for a majority of 78%, with an average delay of 8 days.These results show that symptoms vary from person to person. This also explains why there is no formal rule for all people to present the same clinical signs or the same delay in their appearance. In fact, our study concluded that these clinical signs may persist even after recovery. Among the population surveyed, 68% reported the presence of sequelae dominated mainly by cough, dizziness and arthromyalgia. In this context, the WHO has stated that in a telephone survey of symptomatic adults who tested positive for SARS-CoV-2, 35% of adults had not returned to their usual state of health 2 to 3 weeks after the test and were still suffering from sequelae of the disease [15].

2. Disease management :

Healthcare professionals represent a population of workers at increased risk of developing an infection due to the specific context and content of their professional activity.A very large number of this population included in our study were contaminated with COVID-19. This contamination was mainly detected by a PCR test (45%) and in 13 CT scans were used to confirm the presence of the lesion in % of cases. According to our results, the diagnosis was essentially made by the emergency doctor (41%). In Algeria on 30 April, for the western region, an almost identical proportion of 51.2% of hospitalised patients had a PCR+ test for SARS COV2 [16]. This comparison of healthcare workers in Tunisia and patients in Algeria helped to demonstrate that the PCR test was the most widely used test in North Africa and throughout the world.In our study, only 4% of the infected population required hospitalisation. Treatment was mainly symptomatic (34%). For a majority of 49% of the target population, the infection required an average of 10 days' rest. In a similar survey carried out by doctors at the regional hospital in Nabeul, all the agents were confined to their homes and no hospitalisation was necessary. Treatment was based on Azytromicin, Vitamin C, Zinc and Paracetamol. Progress was favourable in all cases. The average length of absence was 13.7 days, with extremes ranging from 11 to 28 days [11].

During the period of the outbreak, and despite this high rate of infection, there was a remarkable predominance of good compliance with containment (89%). Despite this, a significant percentage of staff had transmitted the disease to their families and colleagues. It should be noted that the mode of contamination for the majority of staff (80%) was intra-hospital, in contact with patients and colleagues. This is compatible with the Nabeul studies, which found that 58 staff (93.5%) were infected within the hospital, 32 staff (51.6%) were in contact with a suspect or positive patient and 26 staff (41.9%) were in contact with a positive colleague [11].

COVID-19 was a pandemic that affected many countries around the world, resulting in a high number of deaths. In our study, 42% of deaths due to the covid_19 pandemic occurred within their families. In Italy in April, around 10,000 healthcare workers were infected and 74 died [17].

Healthcare staff are highly vulnerable to infection by COVID-19 due to a number of factors: asymptomatic patients or patients with atypical symptoms, close relations between hospital staff sharing the same premises, sometimes making it difficult to maintain a proper distance.

III. Protective measures against covid_19 and their application within hospital departments:

Infectious diseases represent an increased risk, first and foremost for healthcare workers, but also for those close to them. This underlines the importance of containment, which is a very important preventive tool alongside vaccination. But despite all these measures, we cannot ignore the possibility of infecting a family member or colleague. Because of this risk of hospital contamination and the fact that containment and vaccination were not the only means of protecting healthcare workers, it was necessary to add other protective measures at hospital level.

1. The distribution and use of protective measures :

In Morocco, only 17.0% of healthcare professionals were satisfied with the resources put in place by the health authorities to carry out their tasks in the response to the COVID-19 pandemic [9]. On the other hand, in a descriptive study carried out in Nabeul in which 430 healthcare workers were questioned, thirty-seven workers (60% of the staff affected) felt that personal protective equipment was not available in sufficient quantities, while 25 healthcare workers (40%) thought that this equipment was poorly used [11]. In our study, 20% of the staff questioned thought that the distribution of protective measures was ideal.Wearing masks is one of the key measures contributing to reducing transmission and saving lives [12]. However, in our study, 70% used surgical masks, whether or not combined with another type of mask (FFP2, washable, protective visor or other). In this context, emphasis was placed on the duration of mask use, which varied according to type. For 42 users of surgical masks, the duration is between 6 and 12 hours, for the FFP2 mask, a number of 24 people used them for a period of between

2 and 6 hours and for the washable mask a concordance was observed between two intervals,

3 people use the washable mask between 6 and 12 hours and 3 use these masks between 1 and 3 days.

2. Hospital habits :

Wearing a well-fitting mask is one of the measures that each of us should apply, along with physical distancing, avoiding enclosed spaces, crowded places and places where contact is very close. As well as ventilating indoor spaces, washing your hands regularly and using a handkerchief or the crease of your elbow to cover sneezes and coughs [18].

In our study, we obtained results that emphasised these measures. Thus, 68% of healthcare workers insisted on barrier measures such as wearing masks, using hydroalcoholic gel, washing hands regularly, and distancing staff from each other. themselves, or with patients or their carers. According to our results, 56 respondents said that their colleagues respected protection procedures. However, a non-negligible 32% of healthcare staff were not interested in these measures and could therefore be a vector for transmission of the virus. Among the observations of the Nabeul study, despite the high level of awareness among the teams, it seems that the most frequent mode of contamination among healthcare staff can be explained essentially by inadequate prevention (no masks worn, no distancing, defective hand washing) [11].

As well as distributing means of protection, the hospital takes responsibility for the spatial and hourly distribution of healthcare staff in order to limit overcrowding, and this was confirmed by more than half the people questioned (56%). The effect of staff rotation on this pandemic is also confirmed by a study carried out in Morocco, in which those who worked more than 40 hours a week were the most affected by EE (43.9%) and PD (20.7%). [9]

IV. Assessment of measures of precautionary measures and impact psychological effects of covid- 19 on healthcare workers :

1. Evaluation of precautionary measures :

Regardless of position or grade, all individuals had a risk of contamination in non-hospital premises (supermarkets, restaurants, etc.). However, for all hospital staff, in addition to non-hospital contamination, there was a high risk of contamination in the hospital's communal premises. According to our results, 32 staff confirmed that preventive measures were followed in these areas. This differs from the results drawn up by Chaouki Mrazguia at the Nabeul regional hospital, where 40 (64.5%) staff did not wear masks or wore them occasionally in these areas. Rigorous hand-washing and correct social distancing between colleagues were only reported in 30 (48.3%) and 42 (67.7%) workers respectively [11]. In the same context, a study was carried out by C. Olivier which also concurred with our results. It was noted that 870/1146 (76%) care workers stated that they had taken part in work meetings, 558/870 (64%) never wore masks or wore them sometimes. In the rest room, during breaks, 1235/1446 (85%) healthcare workers did not wear masks or wore them occasionally [19].

Despite preventive measures, visits from relatives remain frequent as usual, and more than half the population studied agreed with this and would not realise the likely risk of transmission. This represents a danger that could affect the well-being of carers and allow viruses to spread within and outside hospitals. During this epidemic, less use was made of protective measures against covid_19 when treating patients with atypical symptoms. It can therefore be concluded that the failure to comply with barrier measures and to use protective equipment contributed to a large number of cases of contamination among healthcare workers. Our results are identical to those of a similar study by Shneider et al, which found that healthcare workers are highly susceptible to Covid_19 infection due to a number of factors: asymptomatic patients or patients with atypical symptoms, close relations between hospital workers sharing the same premises, and sometimes difficulty in maintaining a proper distance [20].

2. The psychological impact of covid-19 on healthcare workers :

It's true that this covid-19 pandemic is having a major psychological impact. It is causing a great deal of suffering and uncertainty among healthcare workers. In our results, 49% of staff confirmed this suffering. In this context, the Moroccan hospital faced problems in terms of staff demotivation, psychological wear and tear, reduced team morale and professional stress. These results are in line with a study carried out in 34 hospitals in China, which revealed that a considerable proportion of nearly 1,300 healthcare professionals reported symptoms of depression, anxiety, insomnia and stress. [21]

In this respect, a study carried out in Cameron on a sample of 332 healthcare workers showed high scores for anxiety (41.8%) and depression (42.8%). Comorbidity between anxiety and depression was estimated at 14.73% [12]. In fact, this epidemic is having a detrimental effect: overwork, the high risk of being contaminated, and negative repercussions on health professionals, even depression.

3. The covid-19 vaccine :

Vaccination of healthcare workers is a priority in several countries. The availability of personal protective equipment, its correct use, mass screening of contact cases and their isolation remain the key elements in protecting staff and patients. The majority of the population (72%) confirm that, thanks to vaccination, symptoms are less dangerous and serious forms of the disease are less frequent. Even after a correct and complete vaccination, it is important to maintain barrier measures (wearing a mask, hydroalcoholic gel, distancing oneself, etc.). According to a study of Canadian adults, public health recommendations concerning the wearing of masks, physical distancing and frequent hand washing should continue to be observed during the roll-out of vaccination programmes, given the high prevalence of risk factors in the Canadian population. [22]

V. Study limits :

Given that the study involved healthcare professionals from 10 departments of the University Hospital of Gabès, the interpretation and generalisation of the results to all Tunisian healthcare professionals must be carefully discussed, since our study was not addressed to all healthcare professionals working in the hospital.Our sample contained an unequal distribution of men and women. The data in our study was completed by the participants themselves, and this may represent a bias that is common in this type of study. However, this bias was minimised by the anonymous and confidential nature of our study.

RECOMMENDATIONS

As the number of new positive cases of Covid_19 is low, it is advisable to take advantage of this to reinforce the staff of the University Hospital of Gabès (nurses, nurses' aids, intensive care doctors, emergency doctors, technicians) to be ready in case of a new wave. The Covid-19 crisis needs to be managed and those responsible for the failures prosecuted. It is strongly recommended that funding be increased to improve the health infrastructure in order to avoid problems with precautionary measures in the event of other pandemics. We propose to focus on these types of studies in order to highlight the enormous efforts made by healthcare workers during this pandemic.

CONCLUSION

The coronavirus (COVID-19) pandemic spread rapidly around the world from January 2020 onwards, confining entire populations, filling overflowing hospitals with massive numbers of patients with severe forms of the disease, and leading to a dramatic increase in mortality within healthcare services themselves [23].The SARS-CoV-2 pandemic is affecting people around the world, particularly those at high risk of infection, mainly healthcare workers, who are the first line of defence against this pandemic. It raises major concerns about the risk of transmission to patients on the one hand, and to colleagues and family members on the other. This context led us to carry out a descriptive cross-sectional study on a sample of 100 healthcare workers in ten departments at the regional hospital in Gabès, using a questionnaire. This health crisis has had a major impact on our healthcare system. On the one hand, healthcare workers have had to cope with a great deal of pressure and an enormous amount of information in order to manage this pandemic as effectively as possible. Secondly, the distribution of protective measures, which were variable for the ten departments selected, were used according to the needs of the department and the beliefs of the staff, and also depended on the state of the carer (suspect, positive or negative covid19). Our results highlight the physical as well as the psychological impact of workload and individual, social and professional conditions. They should help us to understand the vulnerability of carers to psychological suffering in the face of this health crisis. This difficult period was marked by solidarity between care staff and civilians through moral motivation, education and consolation, and by teamwork and a spirit of collaboration.In conclusion, other measures such as a balanced diet, a well thought-out rotation schedule and psychological support are essential for the prevention and management of COVID-19 in healthcare workers.

BIBLIOGRAPHY

[1] Hongzhou, L., Stratton, C., & Yi-Wei Tang,Y. (2020). Outbreak of pneumonia of unknown etiology in Wuhan, China: The mystery and the miracle. J Med Virol.92:401-2.

[2] COVID-19-Chronology ofaction (2020). https://www.who.int/fr/news/item/29-06-2020-covidtimeline.

[3] Sohrabi, ., Alsafi, Z., Neill, N., Khan, M., Kerwan., Al-jabir, A., .& Agha, R. (2020). World Health Organization declares global emergency: A review of the 2019 novel coronavirus (COVID-19). Int J Surg. 76,71-6.

[4] Chakroun, H., Ben Lasfar, N., Fall, S., Abid, M., El Moussi, A., & Abid, S. First case of imported and confirmed COVID-19 in Tunisia. La Tunisie Medicale 2020;98:258-60.

[5] De Serres, G., Carazo, S., Lorcy, A., Villeneuve, J., Laliberté, D., Martin, R..& Dionne,M. (2020). Epidemiological survey of healthcare workers affected by COVID-19 in spring 2020. 500,12592 -3061.

[6] Perisetti, A., Gajendran, M., Mann, R., Elhanafi, S., & Goyal, H. (2020). Covid-19 extraoulmonary illness-special gastrointestinal and hepatic consideration. Dis Mon. 66(9): 101064.

[7] Chersich, MF., Gray, G., Fairlie, L., Eichbaum, Q., Mayhew, S., & Allwood, B. (2020) COVID-19 in Africa: care and protection for frontline healthcare workers. Global Health.16(1), 46.

[8] Thirumalaisamy, P., Velavan1,2,3* and Christian, G., & Meyer1,2,3*. (2020). The epidemic o f COVID-19.25, 278-280 .

[9] Kapasaa, R ., Hannounb, A., Rachidi , S., Ilungaa , M., Toirambea , S., Tadya, C., & Khalis,M .(2021). Évaluation du burn-out chez les professionnels

de santé des unités de veille sanitaire COVID-19 au Maroc.28, 524-534 .

[10] Prescott, K., Baxter, E., Lynch, C., Jassal, S., Bashir, A., Gray, J.(2020). COVID-19: how prepared are front-line healthcare workers in England? J Hosp Infect. 104(2), 105-5.

[11] Mrazguia, C., Aloui, H., Fenina, E., Boujnah, A., Sonia Azzez,S., & Amel Hammami,A.(2021). L'infection par le COVID-19 chez le personnel de santé à l'Hôpital Régional de Nabeul : épidémiologie et circonstances de transmission. 4(11).

[12] Piere,C., Roger, F., & Ggautier,S.(2021). Anxiety and depression associated with the management of COVID-19 among health workers in Cameroon. 86,131-139 .

[13] Monopoli,G., Marinoa, R., Caldi,F., Fallahi , P., Perretta,S., Cosentinoc,F., .& Foddis, R.(2022). Different clinical results of COVID-19 in male and female nursing staff at a university hospital in Italy. 10, 1775-8785.

[14] Jihane,El., Mekki,N., Deschamps ,L. V.(2021). Recurrence of "COVID toes" after recount with SARS-CoV-2.1(8), 239-A40.

[15] Sakhi, H., Chawki, S., buchard, A., Dardim, K., Boulanger ,C., Mokthar, C., .& Karoui, El.(2020). The long-term effects of COVID-19. 17(5), 269-270.

[16] Hannouna, D., Boughoufalaha, A., Hellala, H., Meziania, K , Lazazi Attiga, A , Aït Oubellia, K., .& Rahal, L.(2020°. Covid-19: Epidemiological situation and evolution in Algeria. 5(1), 2543-3555.

[17] Chersich MF, Gray G, Fairlie L, Eichbaum Q, Mayhew S, Allwood B et al. COVID-19 in Africa: care and protection for frontline healthcare workers. Global Health. 16(1), 46.

[18] Organization World of theHealth. (2022). https://www.who.int/fr/emergencies/diseases/novel-coronavirus-2019/question-and-answers- hub/q-a-detail/coronavirus-disease-covid-19-masks.

[19] Olivier, C., Bouvert, E., Abiteboul, D., Lolom, I., &, G. (2020). Médecin et

Maladies Infectieuses. 50(6),31-199.

[20] Schneider, S., Piening, B., Nouri-Pasovsky,PA., Krüger. AC, Gastmeier, P., & Aghdassi,S. (2020). SARSCoronavirus-2 cases in healthcare workers may not regularly originate from patient care: Lessons from a university hospital on the underestimated risk of healthcare worker to healthcare worker transmission. Antimicrob Resist Infect Control. 9(1),192.

[21] GARNIER,A., VAUCHER,G., BIANCHI,C., KRAEGE,V., MÉAN ,M., CASTIONI,J.,.&VOLLENWEIDER,P.(2020). Organisational impacts and clinical challenges of the COVID-19 pandemic for a university internal medicine hospital service. 16, 869-74.

[22] Finlay, A., McAlister , MD MSc, Tracey Bushnik, MBA, Alexander, A., Leung, MD MSP, & Lynora, S. (2021). Prioritizing COVID-19 vaccination based on prevalence of risk factors among adults in Canada. 193(22), 823-828.

[23] El-Hagea,W., Hingrayc, C., Lemogne,C., Yrondif,A., Brunault,P., Bienvenu,T., Aouizerate, B. (2020). Health professionals facing the coronavirus disease 2019 (COVID-19) pandemic: What are the mental health risks.46(3) 573-580.

APPENDICES

Questionnaire These questions will help us in our study.Please be assured that we are counting on your sincere answers, which will remain accurate and honest.

I. Identification and socio-demographic data :

1) What type are you?

o Female

o Male

2) How old are you?

3) Do you have one or more medical and/or surgical antecedents?

o HTA

o Diabetes

o Heart disease

o Neoplastic pathologies

o Chronic lung diseases

o Or others:

o A history of surgery

if yes

4) What is your workstation?

o Doctor

o Nurse

o Technician

o Worker

5) How long have you been with the company?

o Less than 5 years

o Between 5 and 10 years

o More than 10 years

o Other

6) Which hospital department do you work in?

II. Experience and management of illness :

1. Have you already caught covid_19?

o Yes

o No

2. How many times have you caught this pandemic :

3. What symptoms or signs of the disease did you experience?

o Fever

o Cough

o Diarrhoea

o Headache

o Vertigo

o Or others: .

o Asymptomatic (by screening)

4. How was the diagnosis made?

o PCR

o Quick test

o Scanner

5. The diagnosis was made by?

o The emergency doctor

o The GP

o The referring doctor

o No consultation

o Or other :

6. How long did your symptoms last?

7. What is the deadline for returning to work?

8. Do you still have symptoms or signs of the disease even after recovery?

o Yes

o No

If yes, which ones?

o Arthromyalgia

o Headaches

o Coughing

o vertigo

o or other :

9. Managing the clinical picture required?

o Hospitalization

o Home treatment

10. Have you properly respected the containment?

o Yes

o No

11. What type of treatment have you been taking?

o Symptomatic (antipyretic, analgesic, antiemetic)

o Antibiotics (amoxicillin, azithromycin, cephalosporin, etc.)

o Anticoagulant

o Oxygen therapy

o or other: ....

In your opinion, the mode of contamination was through :

o The hospital

o At home

o Friends and colleagues

o Or other: ....

13. Have you contaminated a member of your family or colleagues?

o Yes

o No

If so, how many people have you contaminated?

14. Have you been vaccinated against covid_19?

o No

o Yes : Type..

15. Do you have any family members or friends who have died as a result of the covid_19 epidemic?

o Yes

o No

III. Protective measures against covid-19 and their application in hospital departments :

1. Is the distribution of protective measures adapted to the needs of your department?

o Ideal

o Average

o Wrong

2. What type of mask do you use when working with patients?

o FFP2 mask

o FFP mask with exhalation valve

o Surgical masks

o Protective visors (face protection)

o Washable mask

o or other :..

3. On average, what is the maximum time you can use a single mask?

Type

4. The safety process in your department insists on barrier measures (wearing masks, hydro-alcoholic gel, distancing, etc.) for staff, patients, their carers and visitors, etc.

o Yes

o No

5. In your department, do your colleagues respect protection procedures?

o Never

o Sometimes

o Often

o Always

6. Time and space allocation within the working environment to limit

is the footprint right?

o Yes

o no

IV. Assessment of precautionary measures and the psychological impact

by the covid_19 in healthcare workers :

1 : no, not at all2 : no, rather not3 : yes, rather4 : yes, completely

	1	2	3	4
The preventive measures applied by healthcare staff are respected in the hospital's communal areas (rest room, cloakroom, refreshment room, etc.)				
For patients with atypical symptoms, the protective measures against covid _19 are respected				
Hospital staff occasionally wearmasks in non-hospital premises (supermarkets, restaurants, etc.)				
During this epidemic, visits from relatives remain frequent as usual.				
This covid-19 pandemic is having a major psychological impact, causing suffering and anxiety. uncertainty among healthcare workers				
Thanks to the effects of the vaccine, symptoms are less dangerous and serious forms are less likely to occur.frequent .				
After vaccination, you need to maintain your barrier measures(wearing masks, hydroalcoholic gel, distancing, etc.)				

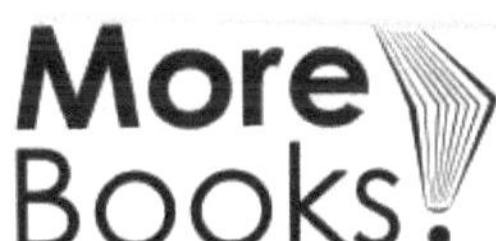

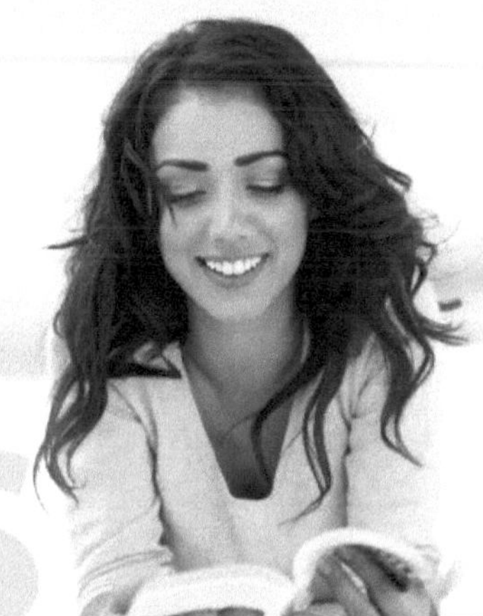

I want morebooks!

Buy your books fast and straightforward online - at one of world's fastest growing online book stores! Environmentally sound due to Print-on-Demand technologies.

Buy your books online at
www.morebooks.shop

Kaufen Sie Ihre Bücher schnell und unkompliziert online – auf einer der am schnellsten wachsenden Buchhandelsplattformen weltweit! Dank Print-On-Demand umwelt- und ressourcenschonend produzi ert.

Bücher schneller online kaufen
www.morebooks.shop

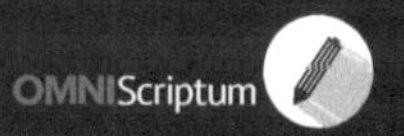

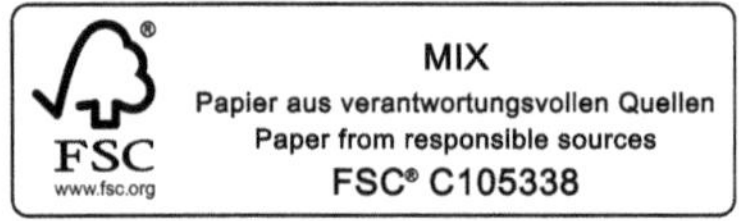

Printed by Books on Demand GmbH, Norderstedt / Germany